T0197052

The Prepared Girl

A book for young girls entering
"The Big Girlz World"

PAMELA EVANS

authorHOUSE®

AuthorHouse™
1663 Liberty Drive
Bloomington, IN 47403
www.authorhouse.com
Phone: 1-800-839-8640

Published by AuthorHouse   07/12/2012

ISBN: 978-1-4772-0552-5 (sc)
ISBN: 978-1-4772-0551-8 (e)

Library of Congress Control Number: 2012908282

CONTENTS

"The Prepared Girl"

This book is not intended to substitute medical advice of doctors. The reader should consult a physician about health concerns and/or symptoms that may require diagnosis or medical attention.

ACKNOWLEDGMENTS

I am very thankful to God for all the wonderful people who helped edit,design,and publish this book.

Thanks to my husband, Leroy who allowed me to pursue my assignment. For all the cooperation, support and encouragement he gave from beginning to end on this project.

Thanks to my children, Destinee, Nikolaus, Christian and Brittani, who make my job as a mom a lot of fun, sometimes a challenge, but most of all a tremendous blessing.

Thanks to my parents, Jack and Sylvia, who gave me the best childhood that I could have and enjoy. It encouraged me to help youth be the best they can be.

Thanks to my grandmother, Minnie, who has always helped me when I couldn't help myself with so many things.

Many thanks to all the girls who gave me the opportunity to teach, train and mentor them in many life and social skills.

Thanks to my entire family, who stepped up and worked individually and as a team to carry the necessary weight for me to fulfill a desire and passion to encourage girls through this informational and fun reading series.

Last, but not least, to all the girls I know as well as those whom I will only get a chance to touch through this book, thank you!

A NOTE TO THE READER

Thank you for supporting "The Prepared Girl" as we give many girls this information to help them be better prepared and give a percentage of our proceeds to girls who need feminine protection during their personal time.

This book was written especially for you. I hope you have as much fun reading it as I had writing it. Enjoy the personal discussions and have fun doing the activities suggested in the back of the book.

Stay encouraged, have fun and enjoy your life as you enter the Big Girlz World, and until we meet again at our next book offering.

INTRODUCTION

"The Prepared Girl" is a keepsake book intended for young girls between the ages of 9 through 15. It is written for girls who do not know what a menstrual period is, those who have heard about it but don't understand it, those who have some knowledge but want more, those who may be afraid of the "first day" experience and those who may have questions they are just too embarrassed to ask. The first 2-3 years of beginning your menstrual period, there are many changes that take place in your body, which may be unfamiliar to you. This book can help you to be better prepared and understand your body and the changes it is going through. You may also learn to be better prepared by the "Shared Experiences" portion toward the back of the book. Never assume your friend's experience will be your experience just because you are both girls.

Because an alarming percentage of girls battle with low self esteem; it is important that girls learn early about some of the issues they may have during this time, and how to handle these issues. Menstrual periods are a perfectly normal event that girls, sometimes as young as 9 years old go through. This book will help teach you what to expect and how to prepare yourself every month.

There is also a menstrual chart to help you keep track of your cycle and a study guide at the back of the book. The study guide can be used to help you discuss this information with your friends' one on one, in a group, with your mom, or wherever you encounter the need. It can also be used as an outline to help older women feel confident discussing this topic with young girls. As you take the time to ask questions and become more informed, you can begin to relax and feel more comfortable for all that will flow in this phase of your life.

Remember, no question is a dumb question. If it crosses your mind, you need to have the guts to ask it because chances are you need to know. Thank you, for making time to read this book and become better prepared for this time in your life!

CHAPTER 1

Menstrual Cycle 101

Every young girl needs to be informed on this subject. You need to know how to properly be prepared during this time each month. It's important to know how to take care of yourself and learn to be aware of your physical changes. Without going too deep into the medical terminology of the menstrual cycle, let's talk about what it is. Menstruation is part of your reproductive system. It signals the onset of puberty, the time when your body begins to physically change. Menstruation is an individual experience of physical and emotional events that occur as your body makes the necessary changes from childhood to adulthood. Now of course this experience does not make you a full grown woman overnight. There are many other areas that require the process of time and development before you become an adult.

One of the first things you need to learn about before your menstrual cycle begins is what type of feminine protection is right for you. For most girls this is what's known as sanitary pads. You'll need to know how often you should change your choice of protection in order to prevent odors and Toxic Shock Syndrome (also known as TSS which is a rare bacteria-caused illness occurring mostly in menstruation women who use high absorbency tampons}. How to dispose of the sanitary product you will be using and not to be ashamed or embarrassed about this time of your life.

Beginning a menstrual period is part of the course of being a young woman. Every girl's menstrual period is different. No one can tell you exactly when it will begin or what you will or will not experience personally. As a girl you need to be informed about this time of your life and the different lifestyle changes you will go through as you age. Girls, who are familiar with what to expect, can be better prepared and less stressed about the unknown. If at any time during your menstrual cycle you experience any of the following, ask your doctor for advice (not your friend}

Excessive bleeding
Missed periods
Unbearable cramps
High fever 102 and up
Nausea and vomiting
Unbalanced emotions (depression or excessive irritability)
Irregular Periods
Blood Clots
Unusual Odor

CHAPTER 2

YOU'RE PERFECTLY NORMAL

Having a menstrual period is a natural part of life and from time to time you may develop symptoms that are perfectly normal. There will be times you'll feel more comfortable than others. Being prepared as best as possible, usually gives you the confidence you need to go with all that will flow. Your menstrual periods, can come regularly or irregularly. Regular means it can come at or around the same time every month or about the same amount of days apart. Usually when regular most girls know whether they will flow heavy or light, and approximately how many days their period will last. For some girls that may mean getting a light flow every month, for others it is regular or normal for them to flow heavy each month during their cycle. Every girl's flow is different. Then there is irregular, which means the cycle doesn't arrive on a regular schedule. One example would be that one month you may begin in 21 days from your last period, the next month or two your cycle may begin after the 28th day. You may flow for 7 days one month and 3-4 days the next month or two. Many girls experience irregular periods, especially in the beginning of starting their cycles. However, you need to talk to a doctor if you're skipping periods or getting them more frequently. There are at times, suggestions a doctor can make as a solution to irregular periods. Also; some girls experience a heavier flow during the time of their menstrual cycle. It has been said that certain foods you eat can cause you to flow heavier. If you find this to be a problem try avoiding excessive sweets and very salty snacks. Girls that are overweight sometimes experience a heavier flow.

Here is a list of a few things that can affect your menstrual cycle and keep it from arriving regularly each month:

Sickness—various illnesses
Physical activity
Crash dieting
Excessive weight loss or gain
Stress
Emotional excitement
Change of environment
Taking medications

Welcome into the big girls world! There will be many things you'll learn about your body as it develops. Whenever, in doubt, don't hesitate to get medical advice from your doctor. Serious and permanent injury to your body can be a result of hormone imbalances, neglect and nutritional deficiencies. Don't ignore your body for fear that something is seriously wrong. Take time to let someone know immediately, so you can get the attention needed to correct the problem. Taking care of your body in every way always benefits you. So start practicing at a young age good hygiene habits, so you won't have many bad ones to correct as you get older. Don't let other girls, or their experiences define if you are normal or not. Tell yourself you are uniquely designed to experience a good life as a Big Girl.

CHAPTER 3

Signs and Symptoms

A few days before your period begins, you may notice some signs. These signs usually give you a heads-up that you need to prepare for all that will flow and that your period is about to begin. However, not every girl gets the same symptoms. There are girls who don't experience any symptoms.

Those that do, may experience cramps, your stomach looking and feeling bloated, backaches, tender or swollen breasts, mood swings, a queasy stomach, an outbreak of pimples, and headaches or fatigue. Wherever you find yourself in these pre-menstrual or menstrual days try to keep track of it by writing it down in a personal notebook or a menstrual chart. Your experience may change from month to month. It is always a good thing to be as prepared as you possibly can. It's no fun being caught off guard, or unprepared.

Fatigue—You may feel sluggish as though you have very little or no energy to do your ordinary task. You may feel like you want to sit down and kick your feet up on a couch or ottoman and keep them elevated for a while. This takes the pressure and tiredness out of your body, and helps you to regain strength.

Bloating—During this time, the jeans you just wore last week may appear to be a little tight due to bloating. You may even feel a little more puffy than usual in your stomach, breasts, hands or face. Don't panic—things will get back to normal in a few days. Just make a note, if this is one of the signs you notice before the flow begins. Most girls find it uncomfortable to wear tight-fitted clothes around this time. If you usually wear pants that fit around the waist, that don't give you room to stretch, you may want to buy a pair that will give you comfort if you experience bloating regularly.

Headaches—Some girls experience slight headache (just enough to annoy you}. There are other girls who experience intense headaches, (sometimes-severe pain that gets your attention immediately, better known as migraines}. Both types of headaches can be related only to pre-menstrual and menstrual days. Again you need to keep track by writing down when the headaches began, how long they last, what area they're in, and if they are severe or faint. Call your doctor with the above information to see if you may use over the counter pain meds or other type of relief prescribed by the doctor. If this is a symptom you experience every month, you may want to be prepared by having the prescribed pain reliever available when and where you need it, for example, in your purse, book-bag, or with the school nurse. Aspirin is not an option during this time of the month because it is a blood thinner that will cause a heavier flow.

Sensitive breasts—Sometimes girls experience more sensitivity than usual around this time. If you notice that your breasts hurt because the bra you normally wear allows them to be bouncy, you may want to purchase a bra that provides a little more support. If your breasts are too tightly supported and the bra is bothersome, you may want to purchase a loose fitting bra for these pre-menstrual and menstrual days.

Mood swings—Some girls experience mixed emotions. During these days you may cry easily, feel like you don't want to be bothered, or get irritated a lot faster. These mood swings are common however, be aware of excessive irritability. Some girls don't experience them at all.

Backaches—For some this is a real" pain in the back", that occurs every month related to premenstrual or menstrual days. You usually feel it in the lower part of your back. There are over the counter—pain relievers you can take with the supervision of an adult. Talk to your doctor about it and get the right kind of medicine. Depending on how much pain you can tolerate, this type of ache could slow you down a bit from your usual routine (at least until the pain reliever kicks in). Most times it's nothing serious, just a throbbing backache that usually goes away after a few hours or a day or two.

Queasy Stomach—Your stomach may feel a little weird. Usually nothing painful unless you are experiencing cramps. This symptom is usually an alert that your period may be arriving soon.

Outbreak of pimples—Sometimes girls notice pimples that pop up on their face, above or beneath their lip, either before, during or after their period. Don't pick at them and don't pop the pimple. Use benzoil peroxide, or a Q-Tip of alcohol to dry it out. Stay away from oily foods during this time and don't see yourself as being ugly. Remember, it's a temporary symptom.

Abnormal odor—If you have a yellowish or brown colored discharge, or an odor that you usually don't have; this would be considered a sign that needs to be brought to the attention of an adult or your physician.

Clots—These may look like clumps of blood that are passed through your vagina. You may notice them when you wipe yourself or in the toilet after urinating. Keep record of their size and of how many and how often you see them. If you see a clot the size of a quarter or silver dollar, this is unusual and needs the attention of a doctor. Also be aware of how much blood you see with them. Use your menstrual chart to keep an accurate record in case you need to give this information to your doctor.

PMS—Pre-Menstrual Syndrome has been said by many to be a "in your mind' type of symptom. Many thought it was something that girls could choose to ignore and it would go away. However, this is a very real disorder. The estrogen level drops during this time and can cause many physical and emotional changes in one's body. Eat fruits and vegetables, avoid caffeine and lots of sugar or excessive junk foods.

Additional Signs & Symptoms

There are other signs or symptoms that you may experience that need medical attention, that include:

- If you are spotting blood at times other than your menstrual cycle.
- If your menstrual cramps are longer than 3-4 days a month
- Excessive vaginal itching
- If you are bleeding for more than a week (7-10 days) with no sign of stopping or decrease in blood flow.
- If your periods come more frequently than 21-28 days a month.

When on your menstrual you can continue to go with the flow of your sport activities. Your menstrual period should not limit you from participating in physical activities unless you are having cramps, or just don't feel like it. Girls who are active before their menstrual are less likely to have really bad cramps. Heavy activity can cause girls to flow heavier, so be aware. You should try to drink more liquids than usual. Remember, menstruation is just one of the many signs a girl gets as a pre-teen or teen that lets her know the body is going through the necessary changes to prepare for womanhood. During this time you must remember your body has become sexually mature enough for you to possibly become pregnant.

Questions and Answers to Help You Get Ready

Q. What does it feel like to have a period?
A. Every girl feels different at this time. Some girls are challenged with symptoms while others aren't.
Q. How will I know when it's over?
A. Your flow will get lighter and you won't need to change your pad as often.
Q. How often should I change my pad?
A. Before you go to bed
   As soon as you awake or after you shower

Every 1-3 hours while you are having a period

Q. What should I do if my period comes and nobody near has a pad?

A. Go to the nearest bathroom, use toilet paper to line your underwear. This will prevent further leaking through until you can get a pad. You also should check the bathroom for a vending machine that provides sanitary pads for a small cost.

Q. How long will my periods last?

A. Usually most girls last between 2 to 5 days (normally no more than 7 days)

Q. When will I get my first period?

A. Many girls get their period between ages 9 to 16 yrs. old.

Q. How much blood will I loose?

A. It varies for everyone but usually the first 3 days will be the heaviest flow, then it should lighten where you need to change pads less often.

Q. What does PMS mean?

A. PMS is short for Pre-Menstrual Syndrome

Q. Is there anything about my period that I should be afraid of?

A. No, there is nothing to be afraid of, that is one of the reasons, it is good to read books like this one and others that are available to prepare you for things you are not familiar with.

Q. What should I do if blood gets on my pants?

A. Don't loose your cool! Almost every woman or girl has had this happen to her at least one time. If you have a jacket, sweater of your own or can borrow your friends, tie it around your waist until you can get to a place to change. If you don't have any type of clothing to cover the spot, ask a friend to walk behind until you get to a bathroom. You can also turn your skirt or pants around where the spot is in the front, and then hide it with your purse, books, or backpack.

Q. What should I use to get the blood out of my panties and clothes? A. Hydrogen peroxide works great! Also some other stain remover products (for clothes} off the shelf in most stores has worked well.

CHAPTER 4

"THE PREPARED GIRL"

During the time of your period, it is a good idea to keep a record of the type of flow you will have from the first day to the last. Every girl's menstrual experience is different. It is good to know what days are usually your heaviest flowing, and if you have cramps or headaches. Having this knowledge about your body helps you prepare ahead of time, so you can go with the flow. One of the best ways to learn what your menstrual cycle is like is to keep good records of your periods on a chart. Here is a sample chart you can use to help you get started.

Keeping this kind of chart will help you take good records of how often your period comes, and if there are any frequent symptoms of headaches or cramps. Most girls get their period in 21-28 days; other girls get their period within 32-35 days. By keeping a record you should begin to see a pattern of your flow. Learning your pattern will help you become more aware of when to expect your period, how long it will generally last, how regular they are of irregular, all of which will help you be prepared to go with the flow each month.

That was then—

In times past, women needed to wear a sanitary belt to keep the pad in place. It was an elastic belt that was worn around the waist, next to the skin. The belt attached to the front and back of the pad, to keep it in place.

This is now—

Today most pads have a sticky strip on the bottom. It sticks to your panty, to help keep the pad from moving around. Some pads also have side wings in addition to the sticky strip. The strip now takes the place of the belt.

You may be familiar with some of the brands commonly used by women or girls you know. Some, if not all, are advertised on TV and in magazines to help girls become more familiar with a certain brand. Though, there a lot of brands to choose from, deciding which one will work for you will not be as difficult as it seems.

There are various types of sanitary products available today and girls have a lot of choices to choose from that can help absorb their menstrual flow. When you begin to shop for pads or sanitary products, you may want to consider purchasing a package for a heavy flowing and another for lighter flowing days. Pads fit on top of your underwear in the crotch area. They have adhesive tape on the bottom to keep the pad from moving around. Some pads have "wings" on the sides of them, which wrap around the edge of your panties. The better the pad is in place, the less chance of blood soaking through and staining your panties and clothes. There are also different brands of overnight pads, super-pads, maxi pads, light-day pads, and panty-liners that are sold unscented and deodorant varieties.

Tampons are also an option. They are a little different from pads. Tampons fit inside your vagina and are a slim tube of absorbent cotton. Tampons, like pads come in various sizes to absorb different types of flows. There are super-absorbent and regular, and tampons with applicators or without. All tampons have a string at one end to use for removing it. You'll need to remember when you put the tampon in, since you can't see how much blood it has absorbed. Changing your tampon every 1-3 hours depending on the type of flow you have is recommended. Never use more than one tampon at the same time. If that doesn't seem to protect you enough use a pad along with it. Tampons can be worn in a pool for swimming. This is one of the big advantages of tampons for those who enjoy swimming.

So now you may ask, ok which one is better? The answer is totally up to you. Some girls like the pad because it's easy to use. You just remove the sticky strip, press it on to your panty and you're ready to go with the flow. Others complain about the pad because you can't go swimming or in the summertime some girls feel icky when it's really hot with a bulky pad between their legs. Many girls like them because they are easy to carry with no bulk in their purse or book-bag. Other girls find them uncomfortable to wear on days they have cramps and still others fear forgetting that they are inside them If it's your first time using the tampon you may want to get permission from your parent first, to make sure you understand how to insert it correctly.

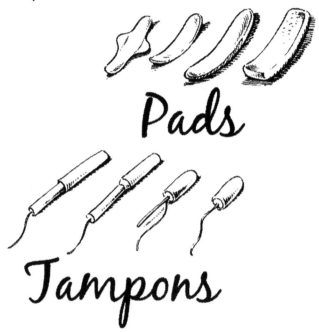

Pads

Tampons

Since both pads and tampons have advantages and disadvantages, many girls make their choice based on personal likes and dislikes, or their need to feel comfortable. Whatever your choice is, a pad or tampon will need to be changed regularly after it has absorbed all the flow it can hold. Pads should be changed every one-three hours. You should get into the habit of changing them frequently before they are soaked, to avoid an odor and blood from soiling your clothes. How often within the one-three hour time frame you should change, will actually depend upon how heavy you flow. Usually when blood becomes exposed to the air, it will begin to cause an odor. You should keep that in mind every time you go to the bathroom.

To keep everything flowing as needed always remember not to throw your pads into the toilet. Wrap them in the paper you take the new pad out of or use some toilet paper and drop it into the garbage can or metal container on the stall wall. Pads that are flushed down the toilet will clog the plumbing and cause big problems. It stops the flow of others being able to use that toilet. Even if you think nobody will know you did it, never, ever, flush a pad down the toilet.

You don't have to feel dirty when you are on your period, if you shower or bathe daily, wear clean underwear changing them every day, and change your pad or tampon often. Most girls say the odor smells like fish. So, if you begin to smell an odor wash yourself, change your pad or tampon then continue with the flow of your regular activities. If you are wearing a tampon don't forget to change it regularly, since you can't see how much it has absorbed. Bacteria can spread and cause problems if a tampon is heavily absorbent and stays in too long. This is called (TSS} Toxic Shock Syndrome. If you have any of the following symptoms while wearing a tampon, remove it immediately and find a pad. Tell an adult and ask to phone your doctor. Some of the symptoms of TSS include:

Diarrhea
Headache
Vomiting
Sudden high fever(102 F or higher}
A sunburn-like rash
Dizziness, fainting
Muscles aches

	1	2	3	4	5	6	7	8	9	10	11	12	13	14	15	16	17	18	19	20	21	22	23	24	25	26	27	28	29	30	31	HEADACHE	CRAMPS
JAN																																	
FEB																																	
MAR																																	
APR																																	
MAY																																	
JUN																																	
JUL																																	
AUG																																	
SEP																																	
OCT																																	
NOV																																	
DEC																																	

Types of Flow: Normal = N Light = L Heavy = H Spotting = S

Headache and Cramps - Intense = I Mild = M

CHAPTER 5

SHARED EXPERIENCES

"It's Official"

I was at home one weekend morning, watching television when I felt something that seemed a little strange. I went to the bathroom and there was blood (bright red) in my panties. I called my mom very loudly, telling her to come quickly. She took one look and said, "Oh no! This cannot be here this soon. I was thirteen years old when I received my period. You are only 11 years old. We just went to the doctor and he said you probably had another year before it would happen." My mom was talking so fast, and then she began to call my dad's sisters to find out when they began their periods. It was as if she was in denial, and could stop it from actually happening until I was 13 yrs old.

She was so preoccupied that she just left me in the bathroom and went to make her phone calls. I had to call her again, "Mom what should I do?" She replied, "Oh honey, I'm sorry, I'm just in shock. I wasn't expecting this to happen so soon and definitely not today." She calmed down and gave me a pad then began to talk to me about things we had already discussed approximately a zillion times lately. Mom took me to the store and showed me the many different shapes and sizes of sanitary pads. She said I should get a small package of two different kinds, so I could decide which was better for me. Once I decided, she told me to be sure I always had enough to last beyond the months demand. She also showed me something known as a sanitary belt used by some women years ago. I said, "No way! I'm not using that thing." She explained that some women felt more secure using a belt, because it held the pad in place. I said, "No way! I'm not using that thing." She explained how it made some women feel a little more secure because it held the pad in place. I chose the pads that had wings, because I was told the wings would hold the pad in place and that was good enough for me. I was so glad my period started on the weekend when I was at home.

This was the beginning of my reality check. Mom told me all about menstrual periods and we discussed things like when we thought it would come, what to do when it came if I was at other places and she wasn't around. The day came, I knew what was happening and wasn't emotional at all that day. I do not remember being concerned about it until the next month, when I really realized what all this meant. This time, I was at home in comfortable surroundings with my support in place, it didn't affect me emotionally. My mom was more emotional than I was. I just thought, "OK, its official now!"

Signed, Relieved

The "In-School" Experience

One Wednesday, I rode the school bus into school as I would any normal day. I was in school for about three classes before going to gym and changing into my gym uniform, when I noticed my panties had blood in them. I had a white discharge every now and again before then, and so I thought, that's what was going on. This time I panicked and immediately felt very uncomfortable. I told my girlfriend getting dressed next to me what happened. However, I did not want her to tell our gym teacher (our teacher was a man}. I was too embarrassed to tell him.

We only had 5 minutes to change and get in the gym before we were marked tardy. I told my friend, if the gym teacher asked where I was to tell him she did not know. I thought he would just think I was taking longer to change, mark me late, and begin class. I was hoping to be able to sit in the locker room until class was over, hoping nobody would notice, except I had forgotten that last week we had picked partners for what we would be doing this week. So the teacher noticed that my partner was alone and asked her where I was. She told him she didn't know, and he asked if I was in school today and she told him yes. He had her check the locker room for me before he would call the office.

When she came in, there I sat waiting for gym to end. I panicked when I heard the teacher talking by the door. As my partner opened the door and called for me, I whispered to her to tell him I was sick and needed to go to the office, I just couldn't explain to my male teacher about my female problem.

The office staff sent me to see the school nurse. She gave me a pad and let me call home so that I could go home and change. This was my "in school" experience.

Signed, Panicked

The "Middle of the Night" Experience

Our school took the seventh and eighth graders on a field trip to one of the local museums. I knew my period would be coming soon, actually any day soon so having heard that exercise was good for you and it helped to prevent you from getting bad cramps. I had increased my exercises. On the day of the trip, we did a lot of walking and standing so after the trip, I was so tired I chose to take a nap and then get my homework done. When I woke up from my nap, I was thirsty so I drank some juice and a big glass of cold water. Since I had taken that nap, I stayed up a little later than usual going to bed around 11:30 pm. Because of all the liquids I drank, I woke up to go to the bathroom about 3:00 am. When I wiped myself, the toilet paper was red. All I could say was, "Uh oh it's here, and I hope we have some sanitary pads. 'What if I can't find them or what if we don't have any, what am I going to do? It is 3:00 in the morning.

This is not really a good time for this to show up. What an inconvenience!"

So as quietly as I could, I began to search the bathroom down the hall for sanitary pads, to no avail. I searched diligently but quietly, so I wouldn't wake anyone by turning on the light or knocking things over.

At this point, now I am wide-awake but sleepy, because I had just gone to sleep at 11:30 pm. I can't find any pads; it's the middle of the night and I didn't want to wake my mom who has to get up for work at 5:30am. I can't go back to sleep so I lay in my bed afraid to move too much. I thought that if I moved too much, the blood would really start flowing, and I did not have a pad on to catch it. What a mess, there in bed, lying on my back very still, trying to fall back to sleep, so I would not be sleepy in school.

My problem was that I sleep every night on my stomach but I thought if I lay very still on my back, I might hear my mom when she woke up for work and she would be able to help me. When I couldn't find any pads, I had to put some toilet paper into my panties to catch the flow. This was my "in the middle of the night" experience.

Signed, Uncomfortable

The "At the Mall" Experience

My friends and I went to the mall on Saturday. We were shopping when one of my friends asked, "Is it just me, or is anyone else really hot?" We all agreed but thought it was only the last store we had gone into. Then it seemed like the temperature was just as hot in the next store, so Victoria suggested we share a locker and put our coats in there. We agreed, split the cost, continued to shop, and then of course we all wanted to eat.

We went to the food court, made our selections and met back at the table to eat together. I said, "I need to go to the bathroom and wash my hands before I eat, I'll be right back." Now remember, we put our coats in the locker. When I used the bathroom, I discovered my period had flowed through my pants. Though the stain was not very big, it was big enough as I had on light-colored pants.

I freaked out and wondered how I was going to get back to the table in this mall on a Saturday with hundreds of people out there. I knew I would see some boys from school as soon as I stepped out the door or before I could get to the table. What was I going to do? They knew I was in here but they did not know what I was experiencing now. They probably thought I ran into someone I knew and was just talking as usual. No one even came to see what was taking me so long to get back to the table and eat lunch.

I was so out of my comfort zone. I beat myself up for putting my coat in the locker. I kept saying, "What were you thinking, stupid? If you had not put your coat up you could have used it to cover yourself as you walked through the mall without worry. Oh, my goodness, why couldn't this have happened before I left home? This was my "at the mall" experience.

Signed, Stressed

The "Over At My Friend's House" Experience

There was a big sleepover planned a month in advance and we received our invitations a couple of weeks before the actual day. Everyone attending had to RSVP one week before the event. The day of the sleepover, there were about 10 girls there. Some I knew, some I did not know, some of the girls were from school, some were from church, and others were relatives. We had fun eating popcorn, nachos, candy, pizza, playing games and so much more.

When it was time for all of us to wash our face and hands, brush our teeth, the last girl was to call lights out! Well, when it was my turn to go to the bathroom I discovered that my period had started? Who do I tell? How can I tell someone, without the other girls finding out? I thought about calling my mom, and then I thought No, she'd come and get me tonight and I'd miss all the fun tomorrow. I had waited too long for this day, which is when I thought, I would just tell my friend's mom she would understand. After all, she is an adult. There was only one problem: I had to get my friend's attention so I could ask her to get her mom for me. Remember everyone was supposed to be in and out of the bathroom like an assembly line, so the last girl could turn out the lights. This being one of my early experiences with this whole menstrual thing had me a little confused about how this was going to work out. My heart was racing as I wrestled with a desire to stay and not miss the fun, but my head had tormenting thoughts of bleeding heavy and flowing through the pad. My mother had explained that I would have to keep track each month to learn about my cycle.

I told my friend that I needed her mom a message from my mom. I then told her mother what had happened and she lovingly helped me. I was no longer confused about who I could talk to about this problem. By the time the lights went out, I was feeling better and when we awoke the next morning, I was ready to have more fun.

My friend's mom called my mom and explained what had happened and told her I was fine. She had taken care of me just as she would have taken care of her own daughter. This was my "over my friend's house" experience

Signed, Confused

The "Big Day" Experience

The school spirit was high today. I had been waiting for this day all week. This year, the cheerleading squad had gotten new uniforms, and I had made the team. Today's game I would have the pleasure of cheering in my new uniform. The game started and we began showing the crowd our new cheers. Jumping and shouting with excitement, we cheered almost non-stop until half time. All of a sudden, I felt something really wet. I got so paranoid, like really nervous. I thought I do not believe this, this cannot be happening to me today of all days. We are in our new uniforms, and this is the first game! Come on, not NOW!

I went to the bathroom to check what this unusual feeling was; only to see what I was hoping would not be there. I rolled a huge wad of toilet paper up and stuffed it into my panties to prevent any leakage to my uniform panties. I went back out to cheer until the end of the game. After the game I got my purse, where I had always stashed a pad for the just-in-case moments like this. This was my "big day" experience.

Signed, Surprised

The "Swim-Meet" Experience

My friend and I were talking and fooling around when the conversation about menstrual periods came up. She mentioned some things about it, and then we both asked, "Where did this come from, anyway? How come boys don't have them?" I am on our school swim team, and we are preparing for a national swim-meet. I am very competitive, and always want to win; coming in first place is always my goal. However, lately I've been noticing when I get my period; I get headaches and feel tired. Sometimes my headaches are faint, but sometimes they are intense like a migraine, and I do not feel like doing anything but lying down. I am really hoping that I do not get my period during the national swim meet. I even had to begin wearing tampons just so I could swim meet. I even had to begin wearing tampons just so I could swim, but I found I really don't like them. But pads in the pool are just not cool; imagine that! This was my "swim—meet" experience.

Signed, Restless

The "Foster Home" Experience

This is to all my sisters who have the experience of coming into a new home with foster parents. These are parents who agree to take care of you when no one else can or wants to.

I had only been in my new foster home for two weeks when my menstrual period started for the first time. I hadn't even developed a relationship with my foster mom, yet. I pretty much just went to school because I had to, came home, did my homework, watched TV, and then I spent some time journaling about my day. I had lived in another foster home before I came to this one. Nobody ever really sat down with me and explained the whole menstrual period to me. I just heard about it in my health education class.

One day, when at home by myself, I went to the bathroom, wiped myself and to my surprise the white toilet paper was marked with a pink color. I didn't get scared. I just thought to myself, I wonder what this is? Without mentioning anything to anyone, I stayed in my room until dinnertime.

My foster mom called my name and said to come and eat dinner. I came reluctantly. You see, I am very shy. I didn't have anything to talk about, and I didn't want to be mean or make her think I didn't want to be there. Actually, I had just been there 2 weeks. So I really didn't know much about her or her home. I certainly didn't know her well enough to discuss my personal business with her (so I thought). The next morning, while getting ready for school I went to the bathroom wiped myself and this time the color had changed from pink to red. I remembered some things taught to me in class. I immediately thought to myself, "Oh no, this must mean my period is here. Just great, what do I do now? I don't know this lady well enough to discuss my personal issue with her. I know what I'll do. I'll just fake being sick; yeah that's it. I'll just tell her I'm sick and I can't go to school."

Then I realized *if I don't tell her, what was I going to use to stop the blood? "Oh, this is just great". She does not know me and I don't know her, and she already has enough to do without me throwing a monkey wrench in her morning. It's not as if I'm*

22

the only girl here. There are four other girls. I wonder what the other girl's did? Maybe I can ask them. Maybe I won't because I don't really know them either, and if I ask them, they will tell her. She might be upset that I didn't tell her myself. This morning is not going well. What should I do? I guess I'd better tell her because if I stay at home and play sick, I'll probably mess up my sheets. I don't have any money to buy some. I can't call my friend because she doesn't have any money either and she has to be in school.

Well, I ended up telling my foster mom my problem, and surprisingly she didn't holler at me. Actually, she was very understanding about it. She gave me a pad, showed me how to put it on, gave me some extras for my book-bag and said if I had any problems to tell the school nurse. If she needs to, she can call her at work. She also assured me that I would be fine. This was my "Foster Home" experience.

Signed, Nervous

Personal Discussions For Girls Only
(Study Guide)

These discussions can help girls learn to be better prepared and allow them to see that they aren't alone. Every girl and woman experiences include uncomfortable and embarrassing days, but we all get through them.

1. What are some of your most embarrassing moments while being on your period? Have you forgotten it, or do you still think about it?
2. Tell about a time you had a thought about being prepared by taking a pad with you, but you ignored that thought. What did you learn about your body?
3. Do you remember the first time you were explained information about menstruation? Share about that time, remembering the place you were at, your age and your level of understanding. How important do you think it is to have someone explain this subject before it is experienced?
4. What are some myths you've heard about—things you can or cannot do when on your period? For example: some say you can't take a bath during your period. Some say you can't wash your hair. Still others say you can't get pregnant the first time. What others have you heard?

Activities To Help You Be Prepared

When You grow up you can give your daughters this book to pass on to their daughters.

1. Some girls can use this book and the topic to begin their own book club possibly calling it "For Girl's Only." Another suggested title may be "Are You Prepared?" It can provide an opportunity for girls to get together in a safe environment both emotionally and physically to begin opening up and discussing issues that are personally for young girls. For girls too shy or embarrassed to volunteer information, you can suggest that each girl write their questions or situation for discussion on paper. The group of peers can then discuss them and generally, they will answer their own questions helping each other make the right decision. This is a great self-esteem builder!

2. Plan a one-night event for young girls entering into this stage of their lives. Make sure to provide a well-supervised comfortable and safe environment for either a girl's night out or a girls' sleepover. Serve their favorite food and drink and play some fun games as you discuss the personal issues they may have begun to experience. Ask each girl you, invite to purchase this book head of time, read it, be prepared to discuss it and look forward to one of the most Fun Girls' Night, they will ever have. Ask them to RSVP only after reading the book. See you at the party: Let the Fun Begin!

3. Have the girls study the words in the glossary individually or in groups. They can use this time to familiarize themselves with the words, spelling, and correct pronunciation. Or they can say the words and give the definition (which is short}. This is a fun way to educate yourself about Yourself. It is always good to be prepared! This is a great game to encourage spelling and health. (You can add to this activity, depending on the ages of the girls}

4. One last suggestion is you can plan a fun formal dinner gathering where the girls dress up and go to a nice restaurant, maybe downtown, and then afterwards go shopping and

sightseeing in the area. You can make this a really fun time by sending invitations as a special guest (VIP} only. Most girls love to go out for a bite to eat and shop! This activity can encourage girls to bond with their peers. The focus should be to inform them of the importance of girls empowering girls. This time can also be used to affirm them in who they are as well as to squash some of the old myths and learn to make good choices as they enter the Big Girls' World. If the parking is too expensive downtown, you can choose a shopping mall most girls have never gone to before. Find a nice restaurant and help them celebrate their coming of age phase at this time. Also, they'll learn how even some of those most embarrassing moments are not meant to be an obstacle to hinder them for life. It's something that happens, forgive yourself then move forward!

These suggestions are opportunities to allow the girls to open up and become informed about their personal body and hygiene. It is an opportunity to dispel myths they might have heard and wondered about but haven't been given the opportunity to ask about. Give them a chance to share their own experiences and gain confidence in the sharing and hearing of each other's experiences and questions. Gaining self-esteem and the knowledge that they are not alone, making it easier to let go of past embarrassments and move forward in a positive manner through this process. If none of these activities interest you, be creative and plan your own. The intended purpose is to help the girls celebrate and understand the transition from childhood to adulthood that they are experiencing at this time in their life.

GLOSSARY

Look at these words and find their meaning, so you can learn more about you!

Female Reproductive Cycle—the monthly cycle, usually 28-5 days in length, that prepares a woman to become pregnant

Menstruation—the monthly flow of blood that occurs when a female egg is not fertilized

Toxic Shock Syndrome (TSS)—a particular group of flu-like symptoms, which can be quite severe, arising from improper use or insufficient changing of sanitary products during the menstrual cycle

Period—the monthly arrival of the menstrual flow

Vagina—the inner channel through which menstrual blood flows; the passage between the uterus and the outside of the body

Hormones—part of the body's regulatory system

Estrogen—a female hormone

Progesterone—a female hormone

Cramps—muscles spasms

MY FIRST TIME

On the lines below, you may want to record your first menstrual cycle experience to share with your daughter or another young girl you care about, to help them with their own first time experience.

_____

_____

_____

_____

_____

_____

_____

_____

_____

_____

_____

_____

_____

_____

_____

_____

_____

_____

_____

_____

_____

_____

_____

_____

ABOUT THE AUTHOR

Pamela Evans volunteers for various organizations that help youth develop for life in many ways. She has been married to her husband Leroy Evans for 27 years, and is a mom of four amazing children ages 26, 18, 16, and 13. Pam has worked with children for twenty four years as a counselor, coordinator, advocate, and mentor in various organizations. Her love and desire to train and encourage and empower youth to respect others, enjoy and celebrate life as they learn to appreciate the joy of giving is a constant passion.

Printed in the United States
By Bookmasters